HERBAL ANTIBIOTICS

Beginners Guide to Using Herbal Medicine to Prevent, Treat and Heal Ilness with Natural Antibiotics and Antivirals

Introduction

The field of herbal antibiotics offers a different sort of ancient world: one that brings a return to old practices, old ideas. Herbal antibiotics offer understanding about the undeniable strength of the plant kingdom. As the forests fizzle and humanity takes to the city streets, knowledge about this plant kingdom fades. Pharmaceutical medicine is found in every cabinet across the world, and miraculous drugs are working to fight undying battles against bacterial infections, against colds, and against serious diseases. However, as scientists develop new synthetic drugs, the bacteria are growing stronger. They're evolving faster than ever. And this evolution and change are creating the disastrous antibiotic crisis. The antibiotic crisis forces society to turn back to what it once knew: herbal antibiotics, in order to avoid the limitations of the synthetic antibiotics.

With herbal antibiotic knowledge, we hold the ability to live optimally. We can eat well to boost our immune system; we can become proactive in our herb picking and utilization. Herbal medicine is empowering because it's about how to live for optimum health. If we begin to understand that there are active healing and immune-boosting compounds in all the vegetables, leaves and herbs that we eat and that the largest part of the equation is keeping our immune system healthy, then we are choosing to be proactive. We don't need to wait until we're ill to think about the subject of healing. Herbal medicine can be there as part of our everyday lives. Should an infection take hold, however, we can then turn to the more potent forms of herbal antibiotics, as outlined in this book.

Herbal antibiotics are bursting with antibacterial, antiviral, and immune system-boosting properties. Each herb outlined in this book maintains a complex structure, one that can beat back against bacteria in a different sort of way than the average synthetic antibiotic. The herbs come from the earth. They've been there, assisting countless generations with their health decisions in past centuries. The rediscovery of these herbs can truly turn the clock back against the antibiotic crisis and create a better, more rounded world: one that turns to the synthetic antibiotics when they are absolutely required, and one that turns to the natural world to seek interior strength and vitality.

Table of Contents

Introduction
Chapter 1: The Reality of Antibiotics
  THE PURPOSE OF ANTIBIOTICS
  HOW DO ANTIBIOTICS WORK?
  THE CURRENT SYNTHETIC ANTIBIOTIC CRISIS
  SYNTHETIC ANTIBIOTIC SIDE EFFECTS
Chapter 2: Herbal Antibiotics: History and Utilization
  PRODUCTION AND PROFITS
  HERBAL ANTIBIOTIC HISTORY
Chapter 3: Immune-System Strengthening Herbs
  GINSENG
  GINGER
  TURMERIC
  GANODERMA
  CAT'S CLAW
  GINKGO BILOBA
  ROSEMARY
Chapter 4: Antiviral Herbs
  ST. JOHN'S WORT
  LICORICE ROOT
  ELDERBERRY
  ECHINACEA
  GARLIC
Chapter 5: Antibiotic Herbs
  CRANBERRY

- TEA TREE
- ARTEMISIA
- USNEA
- OREGANO
- MINT
- CULINARY SPICES

Conclusion

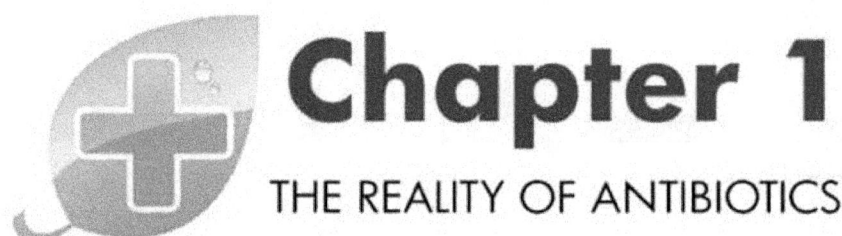

Chapter 1
THE REALITY OF ANTIBIOTICS

THE PURPOSE OF ANTIBIOTICS

Synthetic antibiotics are utilized to treat bacteria-caused bodily infections. They work against fungi, parasites, and bacteria; however they are ineffective in the elimination of viral infections. Each antibiotic fights against either anaerobic bacteria or aerobic bacteria; aerobic bacteria require oxygen to survive while anaerobic bacteria don't require any oxygen.

HOW DO ANTIBIOTICS WORK?

Antibiotics come in a whole range of shapes and sizes and are utilized for a variety of medical purposes. Generally, however, synthetic antibiotics work in one of the following two ways.

1. They work as a bactericidal. A bactericidal eliminates bacteria completely. It works to alter the bacteria cell on either a cell wall level or an interior cell DNA level.

2. They work as a bacteriostatic. A bacteriostatic forces the bacteria to stop multiplying.

THE CURRENT SYNTHETIC ANTIBIOTIC CRISIS

The media is blaring it across all speakers. The world is in a middle of an antibiotic crisis. Bacteria are increasingly resistant to the synthetic antibiotics doctors throw at them, resulting in a new ultimate affront of bacteria. As each new bacterium evolves, new synthetic drugs must be developed to compete with them. How, exactly, does this happen so quickly? Essentially, bacteria are some of the most adaptable organisms on the planet. Their reproductive rate is only twenty minutes—while humans wait a full twenty years, usually, before reproducing. Furthermore, each reproduction results in a new evolution. These new strains of bacteria can also teach other strains of bacteria how to build themselves up against other strains. And how long can this go on? The medical world understands that the days of synthetic antibiotics are coming to an end. People must begin to prepare themselves for this abrupt future.

One of the reasons this antibiotic crisis emerged is because medical doctors overused and over-diagnosed seemingly "miracle" antibiotics for several years. Penicillin, the miraculous antibiotic that annihilated countless diseases in the mid-20th century, provides a prime example of this over-diagnosis. It was discovered in 1942; however, less than a half-century later, forty million pounds of penicillin was utilized in the United States every single year. Today, over sixty million pounds of penicillin is used every year, rendering itself ultimately useless in the coming century because of its over-usage. Bacteria, as aforementioned, can formulate itself against this onslaught of antibiotic. Soon, this over-usage of penicillin will surely result in tragedy as the bacteria work against the drug.

Furthermore, research shows that synthetic antibiotics enter and exit the body generally unchanged. This means that they work through the digestive system and into the greater "water" of the world without altering. After the water cleanses itself via the water table processes, the water still maintains low levels of this antibiotic "waste." Therefore, even as people drink regular water, they are still building a small resistance to their antibiotics. Ultimately, these antibiotics won't work as efficiently on these people because the bacteria in their bodies already understand how to work against it.

Of course, stemming the usage of synthetic antibiotics in the current culture proves difficult with the rush-around mentality of society. People want to eliminate their illnesses immediately, and who can blame them? No one wants to feel terrible. No one wants to miss out on life because of sickness. Synthetic antibiotics are invaluable because they act quickly. They are powerful in all life-threatening illness situations. However, society must stem their usage of these synthetic antibiotics and reserve these antibiotics for life-threatening scenarios. They must limit the antibiotics' recent attack on the environment, as well, via the water supply. Furthermore, these antibiotics must be eliminated in their usage to build strength and health in factory farm animals. The synthetic antibiotics do have a purpose, and they were created for a reason. However, these reasons have been stretched to cover nearly everything in the world, rendering them nearly useless in the years to come.

Furthermore, with each dosage of the synthetic antibiotics, people's immune systems immediately begin to break down. The immune system is an incredible mechanism that initially allows a person to refute attacks from bacteria slowly. However, synthetic antibiotics actually enter the body and kill both good and bad bacteria. They kill, for example, the undeniably important flora from the digestive tract. This elimination of the flora can result in things like yeast infections and un-due upset stomachs. Remember that the body requires a continued defence against constant attacks, and eliminating these good bacteria initially creates a bland environment in which one can become immediately more ill.

Synthetic antibiotics require a specific "course" for people to follow. When, for example, a person begins an antibiotic but does not complete the designated course, the person leaves a few hefty bacteria alive in his system. These left-over bacterium actually work to regenerate to the "next generation" of surviving bacteria, thus having the ability to be resistant to the very antibiotics that once could have taken them down.

The antibiotic crisis creates a vicious cycle of stronger and stronger drugs, of stronger and stronger bacteria, and of weaker and weaker immune systems. People must begin to look to the ultimate rewards of utilizing herbal antibiotics in order to escape from the cycle and fuel themselves toward better overall health.

SYNTHETIC ANTIBIOTIC SIDE EFFECTS

Synthetic antibiotics are becoming increasingly ineffective against the realm of bacteria. However, antibiotics further push several unfortunate side effects that can be avoided with the usage of antibiotic herbs.

1. Vaginal Yeast Infection

As mentioned in the previous section, the usage of synthetic antibiotics actually eliminates all the "good" bacteria from a person's digestive tract. As the good bacteria slides away from the digestive tract, the yeast can begin to grow rampant in the vaginal and digestive arenas. This imbalance between bacteria and yeast results in the yeast infection. A yeast infection includes embarrassing and uncomfortable elements like redness, swelling, itching, and a burning sensation in the vaginal area. A 2013 antibiotic study showed that twenty-five percent of all women who took synthetic antibiotics actually developed yeast infections.

2. Nausea, Vomiting, and Diarrhea

Each digestive tract must maintain a healthy dose of good and bad bacteria in order to create proper digestion. Synthetic antibiotics disrupt this balance and cause diarrhea. According to a recent study, approximately fifteen percent of all antibiotic users have antibiotic-related diarrhea.

3. Medication Interaction

Society's constant clamour for more and more medications can ultimately lead to interactions between the various medications. Side effects that result from these interactions include headaches, stomach aches, and further serious health problems. Furthermore, other synthetic antibiotics can actually reduce the body's ability of proper functioning. An example of this is found with the usage of some oral contraceptives. Other synthetic antibiotics can hinder the contraception and result in an unplanned pregnancy. It is important that people keep a constant dialogue with their doctors about the medications they take to ensure proper functioning.

4. Undue Hypersensitivity or Allergens

Several patients report having allergic reactions to the synthetic medications they take. According to a 2011 study, approximately thirty-two percent of drug allergy cases were caused by antibiotics. These allergens are seen physically on a skin level with the appearance of rashes or hives.

Other, rare side effects include: kidney stones, sun sensitivity, feelings of loss of hearing, and occasional abnormal blood clotting.

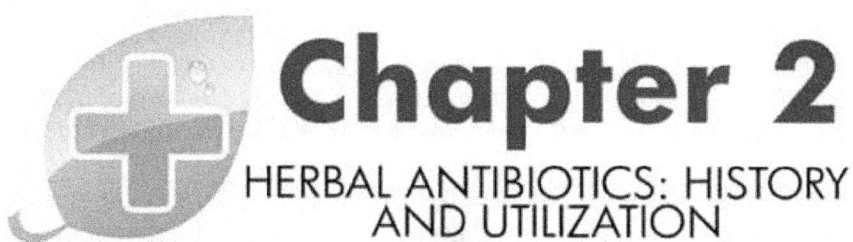

Chapter 2
HERBAL ANTIBIOTICS: HISTORY AND UTILIZATION

Herbal antibiotics, on the other hand, hold none of the negative properties of the average synthetic antibiotics. But why, exactly, doesn't the body's harmful bacteria resist to the antibiotic properties of the herbs? Certainly, if the bacteria ultimately resist the antibiotic nature of synthetic antibiotics, they'll resist the nature of the herbal antibiotics. Won't they?

The supreme difference between the herbal antibiotics and the synthetic antibiotics is in their evolution. Plants and herbs have learned to survive several million years of disease-causing fungi, viruses, and bacteria. The various plants and herbs have developed a systematic complexity, one that is overwhelming to the average bacteria. Synthetic antibiotics don't have such a complex structure. Instead, they operate with single all-mighty ingredients that eventually underwhelm the bacteria and are basically "eaten up" with the incredible evolutionary abilities of the bacteria.

With the ingestion of these herbs, the body takes in all the complexity of the herbs and plants. Because of this complexity, the herbs hardly ever simply kill the bacteria. Instead, they work to strengthen the immune system; they cleanse the blood and improve the organ functionality. Herbs, therefore, are not attack-oriented. Instead, they build the body to greater heights to allow it to defeat the organism itself, thus allowing it to learn how to defend and thus perpetuate strength for future attacks.

PRODUCTION AND PROFITS

The utilization of one ingredient in the normal synthetic antibiotics is a result of patent and financial purposes. Modern researchers work to understand one single, strong ingredient and then claim it to grab all necessary financial rewards. Since the first utilization of the synthetic pain killer, morphine, in 1805, society's look toward herbal remedies has fallen dramatically. However, it's important to note that people in second and third-world countries often look toward herbal antibiotics in order to heal themselves. Without the "rewards" of a first world society, they find their strength growing from the earth.

The modern medicine movement is creating a fearful culture, one that looks to the future of lack of effective synthetic antibiotics with feelings of loss. This culture looks to the herbal antibiotic ideas with cynicism; after all, doctors and in-depth surgeries and modern tools are the norm. Documentaries and TV dramas find their basis in hospitals. Mixing a few herbs in the garden can be deemed a bit medieval, a bit out-of-touch. However, recent studies have shown oregano oil to be stronger than one of the strongest antibiotics in today's hospitals, Vancomycin.

HERBAL ANTIBIOTIC HISTORY

The history of herbal medication orients itself in Europe, where the portrait of women hovering over boiling pots of herbs was quite a norm. The thirteenth century, however, displaced these women with graduating medical doctors. In fact, the French word for herb, "drogue," was essentially utilized for the chemical word, "drug," in the later centuries when these same medical doctors began cultivating the herbs to actually develop synthetic antibiotics.

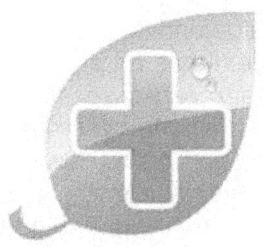

Chapter 3
IMMUNE-SYSTEM STRENGTHENING HERBS

The immune system is a humming machine of complexity. It maintains the essential ability to remember past diseases and defend the body from falling once more to stress and illness. Furthermore, it has an enhanced communication system that brings the necessary response to the triggered reaction of an infection or a wound. The immune cells create the proper secretions that further boost immune "fighter" cells. However, the body's immune system can falter, resulting in days of sickness. Work for a stronger immunity by eating well, resting well, exercising, being out in the sunlight, and reducing your levels of stress.

As aforementioned, synthetic antibiotics can actually hinder the immune system, refuting the good bacteria in places and allowing further growth of harmful bacteria in a weak immune system. Look to the following immune-boosting herbs in order to sustain the immune system. The immune system strengthens itself via the support from the stomach. It is well-documented that malnourished people throughout the world are at greater risk for disease. Therefore, it's important to nourish ourselves well with the following herbs.

GINSENG

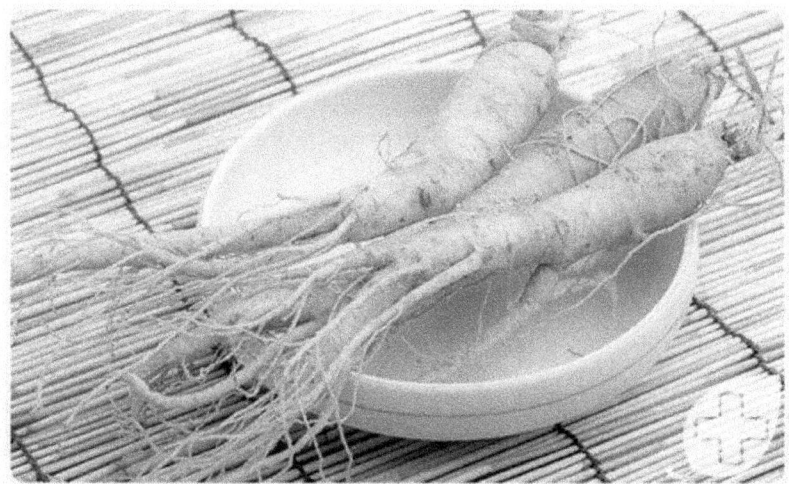

Ginseng is found all over the world in several different varieties. Panax ginseng, or Korean ginseng, is perhaps the most common. Its main ingredient, ginsenoside, holds anti-inflammatory and anti-cancer attributes. It works to boost the immune system and heal the cells from any free radical damage from either the environment or poor dietary choices. Furthermore, it's been known to fight back against diabetes.

Asian Ginseng Chicken Soup

Note: The following recipe is excellent in the repair and healing of the spleen and stomach as well as boosting the body's immune system. It utilizes the root filaments, the small strings that fall from the main root of the ginseng plant.

Ingredients:
4 chicken legs
5 red dates, pitted 10 grams ginseng filaments 2 slices ginger root 1 tsp. salt
6 cups water

Directions:
Begin by cutting the chicken legs into two pieces. Bring a pot of two cups of water to a firm boil and then poach the chicken in the water for thirty seconds. Afterwards, remove the chicken from the boiling water and drain the chicken.

To the side, place the chicken, ginseng, dates, ginger root, and the water together in a safe, heat-able bowl. Steam the bowl's ingredients together in a steamer or in a wok over boiling water. Continue to heat it for two hours, and consistently renew the water supply as the water evaporates. After two hours, remove the soup from the heat and serve warm.

GINGER

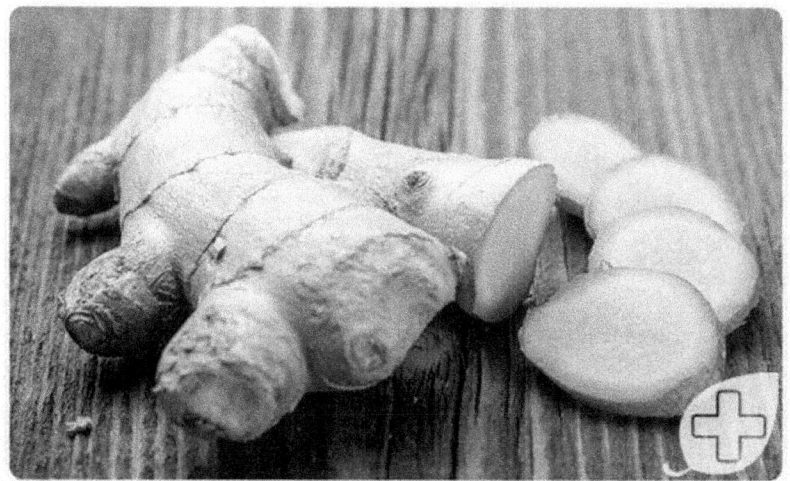

Ginger, a root with a hard, ugly exterior, is pulsing with anti-inflammatory properties. Ginger actually works to eliminate the reaction to certain inflammatory-causing genes. Inflammation is perhaps the number one killer, the ultimate cause of all bodily diseases like cancer, diabetes, and the common cold. As one reduces cellular inflammation, one is actively refuting future sickness. Furthermore, ginger works to fight blood clots, high cholesterol, and cardiovascular disease.

Ginger Chilli Tuna Tartar

Ingredients:
2 onions
1 lb. tuna
1-inch ginger root
1 hot red chilli
6 tbsp. soy sauce
1 tbsp. honey
2 tbsp. sesame oil
Juice from 1 lime
4 slices Ciabatta bread ***Directions:***
Begin by preparing the tuna. Slice and dice the tuna, removing all dark portions of the bloodline. Place the prepared tuna in a large bowl and keep the fish chilled.

To the side, prepare the vegetables. Slice and dice the red chilli, onion, and ginger root. Add the onion, chilli, and ginger to the tuna bowl and stir.

To the side, stir together soy sauce, lime juice, honey, and sesame oil. Pour this mixture in with the tuna, as well, and continue to mix.

Toast each piece of Ciabatta bread in either a toaster or in a griddle. Serve the tartar on the toast, or directly to the side of the toast, for a delectable experience.

TURMERIC

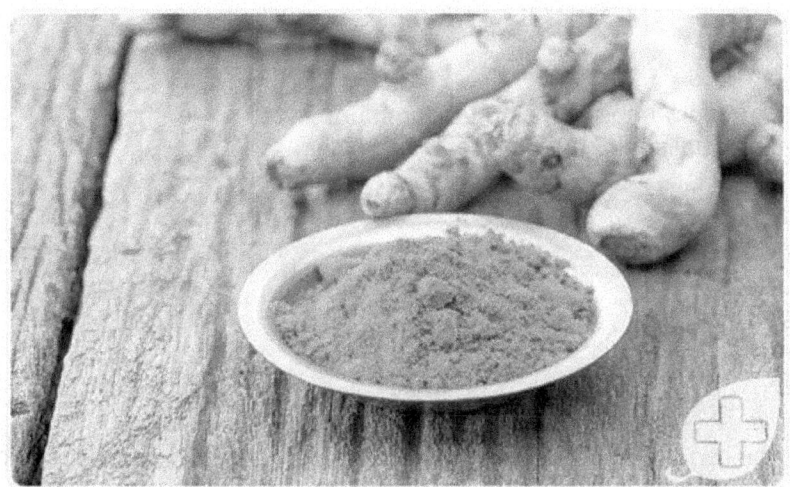

Turmeric is an ancient Indian herb that contains curcumin. Curcumin is rich in antioxidants, which refute inflammation caused by free radicals in the body. Furthermore, it soothes the stomach by boosting the flow of bile and works against bacterial infections. Turmeric stimulates the body's adrenal glands in order to boost the hormone that decreases signs of interior inflammation. Further studies show that turmeric further protects the liver; therefore, the toxins gleaned from heavy drinking can be stemmed with the usage of turmeric.

Ginger and Turmeric Tea

Eliminate interior aches and boost the immune system with the rejuvenating qualities of both turmeric and ginger.

Ingredients:
¼ tsp. ground turmeric ¼ tsp. ground ginger
¾ cup water
1 tbsp. soy milk
1 tsp. honey

Directions:
Begin by boiling the ¾ cup water in a saucepan. Pour in the turmeric and the ginger and reduce the heat to low. Allow the water and ingredients to simmer for approximately ten minutes. Afterwards, pour in the milk and stir well. Strain the mixture into a tea cup and add the honey for a bit of sweetness.

Western Wonder Turmeric Tofu Scramble

Ingredients:
1 tbsp. olive oil
14-16 ounces tofu
½ cup red pepper
¼ cup white onion
¼ tsp. coriander
½ cup Anaheim pepper ¼ tsp. garlic powder ¼ tsp. cumin
1 ½ tsp. turmeric
½ tsp. salt

Directions:
Begin by removing the tofu from the packing and place it on a dry dish towel. Blot at it with paper towels until the extra water is removed. Next, place it in a bowl and utilize a fork to mash it up. The tofu should be crumbly.

To the side, heat up the olive oil in a skillet on medium. As it heats for a moment, prepare the red pepper, white onion, and the Anaheim pepper by slicing and dicing. Toss them in the oil. Cook for a good four minutes, stirring occasionally.

Afterwards, add the cumin, coriander, garlic powder, and salt to the pepper and onion mixture and continue to stir for one minute. Add the smashed-up tofu and the turmeric. Cook for about two more minutes and season with salt and pepper, if desired. This recipe can be eaten on its own or served in warmed tortillas with avocado garnishes.

GANODERMA

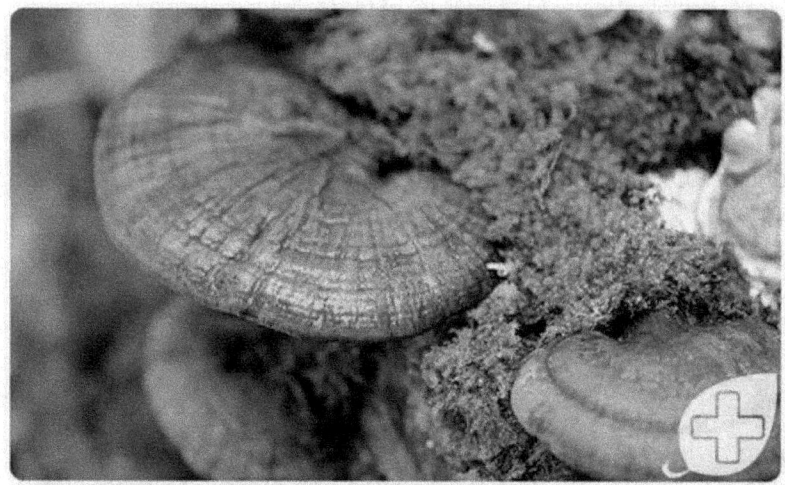

This Asian-based herb is a bitter mushroom. It was utilized in Chinese medical practices for several centuries, and recent studies show that the herb boosts immunity and fights initial signs of cancer. It holds antioxidants, as well, which reduce bodily inflammation while providing interior relief. Look to this herb especially when hoping to reduce pain from urinary tract infections. The best way to utilize ganoderma for its health properties is to drink reishi mushroom tea.

Reishi Mushroom Tea

Ingredients:
5 grams dried Reishi Mushrooms (try Mountain Rose Herb brand from local health food store)
3 cups water

Directions:
Breaking apart ganoderma is incredibly difficult; many report breaking their coffee grinders or food processors in the process. Utilize whatever you have. Try a heavy blade or simply meticulously, with fingers. Alternately, buy a pre-cut bag of reishi.

Bring the three cups of water to boil. Add the mushroom pieces to the boiling water and reduce the heat of the stovetop to low. Allow the water to simmer for a full two hours.

Afterwards, strain the water and set the tea to the side. Allow the tea to cool for a few minutes prior to drinking. Note: the tea will keep for up to three days in the refrigerator.

CAT'S CLAW

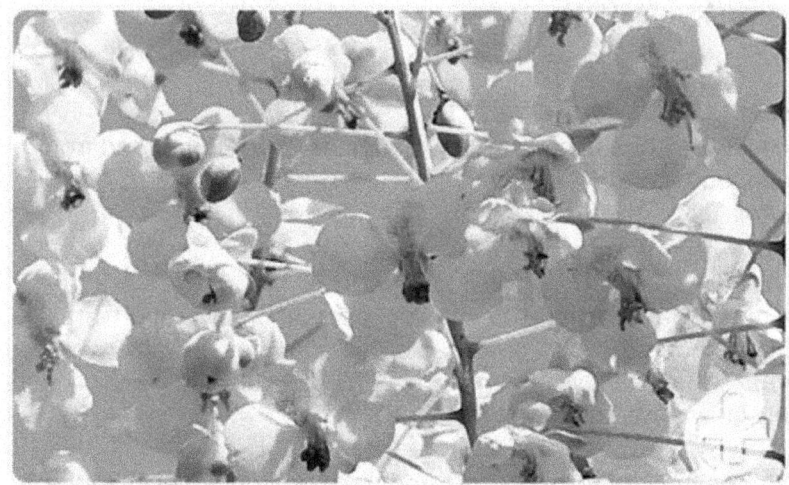

Common utilization of Peruvian herb, Cat's claw, is to heal stomach issues. However, recent use has been shown to boost the immune system. It stimulates the immune system, allowing secretion of greater amounts of fighter cells. Furthermore, cat's claw contains oxindole alkaloids, which boosts the body's ability to swallow up and eliminate bacterium and viruses.

Immunity-Boosting Antiviral Tea

Note: this immunity-boosting tea also contains chuchuhuasi, which has been known to reduce people's joint pain.

Ingredients:
1 tsp. vanilla
2 tbsp. Goji berries
½ tsp. Bercampuri
1 tbsp. cat's claw
1 ½ tbsp. chuchuhuasi

Directions:
Begin by boiling two litres of water in a sauce pan and then placing all the ingredients in the hot water. Allow the water to simmer for a full ten minutes on low. Afterwards, steep the ingredients and serve warm.

GINKGO BILOBA

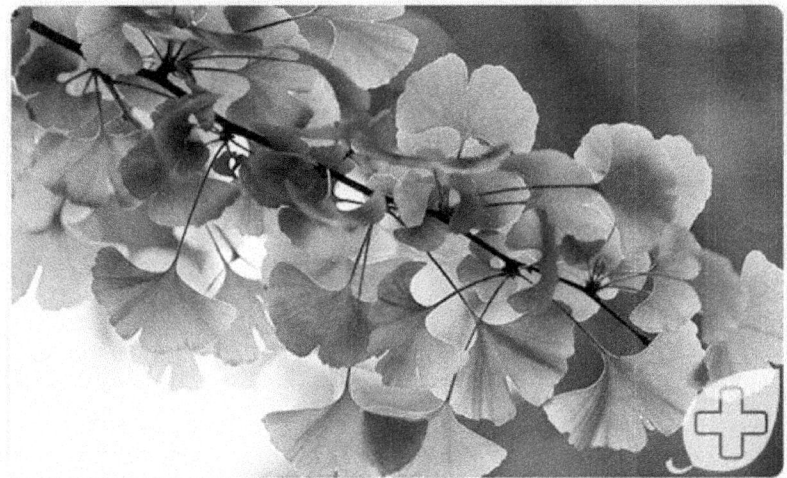

The free radicals pulsing in the body from the exterior environment or improper nutrition find their end days with the utilization of the herb ginkgo biloba. The leaves of the gingko biloba hold bilobalides and ginkgolides that work to refute these free radicals and reduce inflammation. Furthermore, these properties have shown to reduce harm caused by radiation. Recent research shows that the herb neutralizes the free radicals that cause cell death as a result of radiation; furthermore, gingko reduces brain cell damage by approximately fifty percent.

Ginkgo Herbal Tea

Ingredients:
1 tsp. dried Ginkgo biloba 1 cup water ***Directions:***
Begin by boiling 1 cup of water. When it begins to boil, pour in the dried herbs. Readjust the stovetop to a low setting and allow the water to simmer for twenty minutes. Afterwards, strain the water and allow it to cool for a moment in a coffee mug. Drink while still warm.

ROSEMARY

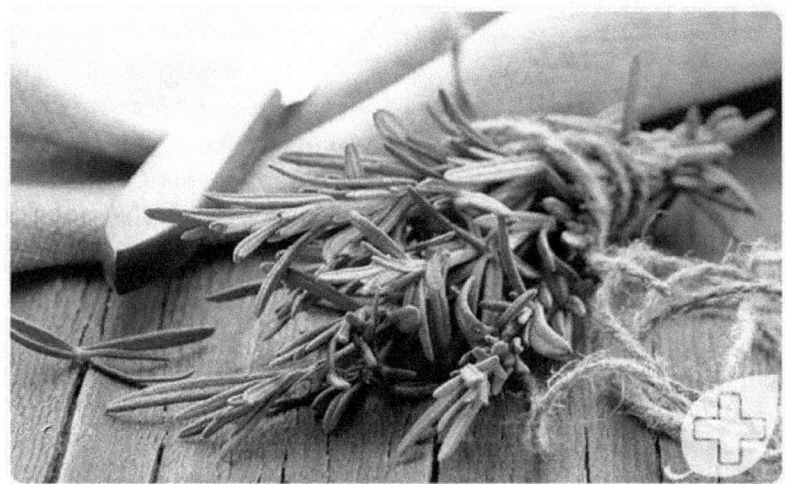

The Ancient Greeks and Romans long enjoyed the beautiful aroma and evergreen nature of this Mediterranean plant. The rosemary plant boosts the immune system and increases blood circulation, thus allowing oxygen to arrive to body cells more quickly. The brain finds itself strong, with essential concentration. Furthermore, this increased blood flow improves digestion and decreases asthma attack harshness.

Raz-Matazz Rosemary Grilled Sweet Potatoes

Ingredients:

6 huge sweet potatoes

½ cup fresh rosemary leaves ½ cup olive oil
1 tbsp. pepper
1 tbsp. salt

Directions:

Begin by preheating the oven to 325 degrees Fahrenheit. Chop up the potatoes lengthwise into fry-like components. Place the fry-like wedges on a baking sheet and drizzle the sweet potatoes with 1/3 cup of olive oil. Afterwards, sprinkle the fries with rosemary, salt, and pepper.

Place the baking sheet in the oven and turn the fries after ten minutes. Allow the fries to continue to cook for twenty minutes more.

Prior to serving, drizzle the sweet potatoes with the remaining olive oil.

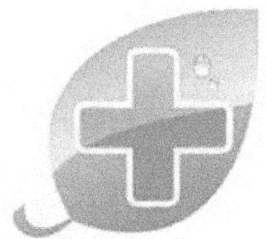
Chapter 4
ANTIVIRAL HERBS

As aforementioned, synthetic antibiotics have no effect against the face of viral infection. In fact, the utilization of synthetic antiviruses can actually breakdown the immune system and result in greater lengths of illness. Viral infections are generally caused in the fall and spring months, when people's immune systems are a bit low, a bit weak, and susceptible to attack. Viruses are small pieces of nucleic acids that boost themselves into people's living, healthy cells; they alter the interior of people's cells to create additional viruses. While it's important to digest healthy foods and drink herbs in the form of tea in order to eliminate chances of attack, there are several natural treatments that refute these viruses and hinder the length of the subsequent illness.

ST. JOHN'S WORT

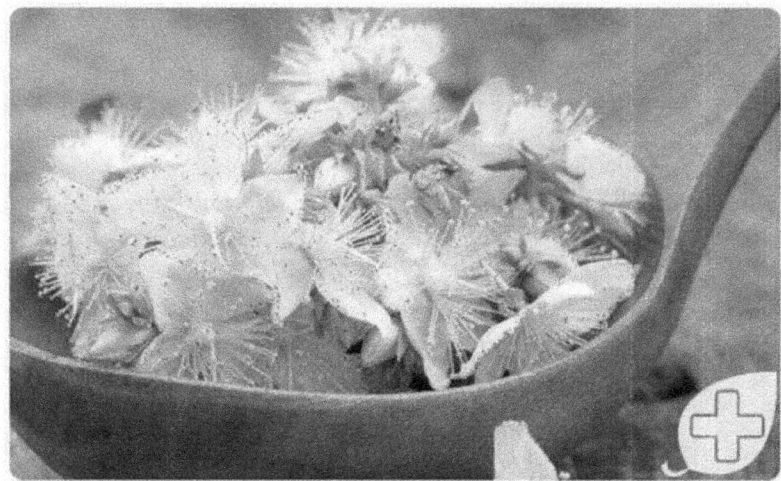

St. John's Wort has been utilized over several centuries to treat sadness and depression. It has been further utilized to assist with rapid cut and wound repair. Recent laboratory studies show that St. John's Wort is pulsing with antiviral properties; it can work against influenza, HIV, and herpes. The pseudohypericin chemicals that reside in the St. John's Wort attack the DNA material of the viruses and they leave the DNA material of the bodily cells alone.

Wound Disinfection

Ingredients:

1 2/3 ounces St. John's Wort Flowers ½ cup 100-proof alcohol

Directions:
Begin by pounding the flower with a mortar and pestle until it's powder-like. Place the herb in the 100-proof alcohol, sealed, for a full ten days. Afterwards, strain the alcohol. Utilize the alcohol for the disinfection of wounds and the relief of frostbite. One can further use it to relieve inflammation.

St. John's Wort Medicinal Tea

Ingredients:
2 tsp. dried St. John's Wort
1 cup water

Directions:
Begin by boiling the one cup of water in a saucepan. Afterwards, pour the dried herbs into the water and put the stovetop on low. Allow the water to simmer for twenty minutes prior to straining the water. Prior to drinking, one can administer a bit of honey to the beverage for desired sweetness.

LICORICE ROOT

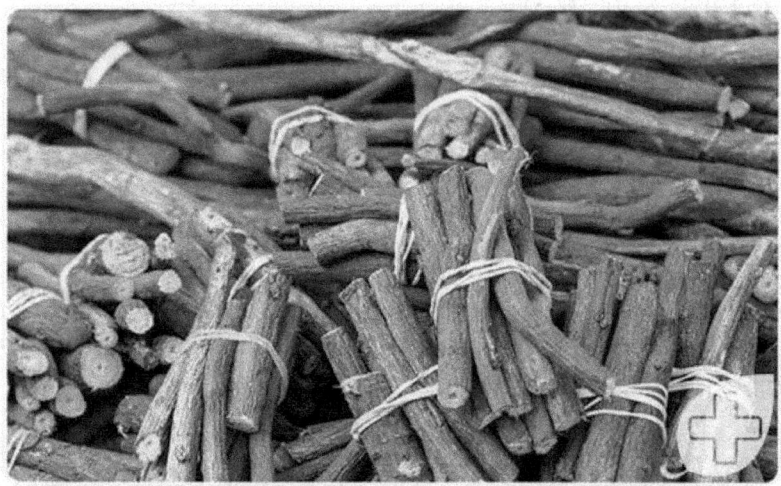

A recent SARS epidemic activated a hunt for proper antiviruses in order to eliminate the disease. German researchers found that the compound in the root of the licorice plant, glycyrrhizin, was truly effective in treating the disease. The root was not toxic to the other bodily cells, and therefore did no greater damage. The interior compound of the root, glycyrrhizin, actually reduced the rate of replication of the SARS virus, in this case; it further inhibited the virus' ability to break into the bodily cell walls and alter the cell neural content. Furthermore, licorice has been noted to halt the synthesis of HIV cells in a lab setting. Because HIV is a viral infection, the understanding of this great herb is incredibly important moving forward.

Licorice Root Tea

Ingredients:
¼ cup licorice root
2 quarts of water
1 fresh ginger, sliced

Directions:
Begin by boiling the two quarts of water on high. When the water has begun to boil, place the licorice root and the fresh ginger in the water. Make sure they've been chopped into the smallest possible pieces to maximize their flavour. Place the stovetop on a low setting and allow the water to simmer for thirty minutes. Afterwards, remove the water and strain it. Drink warm. The tea will keep in the refrigerator for about three days.

Licorice and Coriander Meat Sauce

Ingredients:
1 ½ pounds pork
8 mushrooms
½ cup shrimp
1 cup shallots
½ bunch coriander leaf 16 garlic cloves
1 tsp. licorice
1 tbsp. sugar
½ cup white wine
2/3 cup soy sauce

Directions:
Begin by preparing the mushrooms. Soak the mushrooms in hot water with a cover overtop of them for about an hour. Afterwards, place the mushrooms on a cutting board and mince. Reserve 1 cup of the soaking mushroom water, and pour the rest away.

Heat a wok on medium-high heat to the side. Add in a quarter of the pork. Stir the pork for about three minutes. Next, add the chopped shallots and stir for an additional three minutes. Next, add the shrimp, the cilantro, the mushrooms, and half of the garlic cloves.

Transfer the mixture to a bowl.

Next, place the wok on high heat. Add the remaining pork and continue to stir fry for about five minutes. Add the sugar, 2 tbsp. of the soy sauce, and the licorice. Stir until the meat is completely brown.

Now, pour the bowl-mixture back into the wok. Add the 1 cup of left over mushroom water and the remaining soy sauce along with the white wine.

Bring the mixture to a boil. Add the remaining garlic and salt and pepper to taste. Allow the mixture to simmer for thirty additional minutes. Afterwards, serve the meat sauce with rice for full flavour.

ELDERBERRY

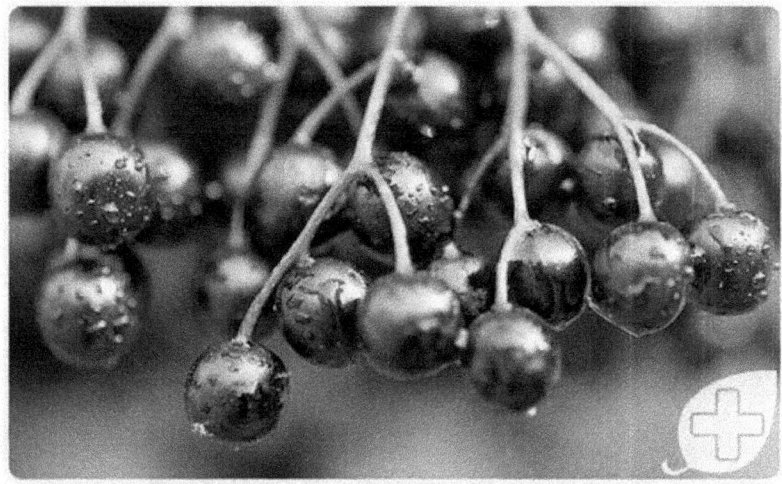

The black elderberry is world-renowned as one of the world's most antiquated and essential remedies. The elderberry finds its particular niche in the fight against meddlesome influenza. A recent double-blind trial has shown that the elderberry herb creates essential assistance. An enhanced immune response is created from the usage of the elderberry, resulting in up to a four day decrease in the length of the influenza. The elderberry properties bind to the small bits of protein that reside on the exterior of the birus cell. Flavonoids in the elderberry further work to protect bodily cells from greater attack. Elderberry has been shown to reduce the re-creation of all four strains of the herpes simplex virus; it has further been found to decrease infection caused by HIV.

Furthermore, its antiviral properties offer a sound relief from the constant flu side effects. It loosens the phlegm and mucus clogging the lungs and the nose, resulting in greater strength and feelings of vitality.

Elderberry Cold and Cough Syrup

Ingredients:
2 tbsp. ginger root
2/3 cup elderberries
3 cups water
½ tsp. cloves
1 tsp. cinnamon
1 cup local honey

Directions:
Begin by placing the water in a saucepan and adding the ginger, elderberries, cloves, and the cinnamon. Bring the mixture to a boil. Afterwards, cover the mixture, reduce the heat to low, and allow it to simmer for forty-five minutes. Remove the saucepan from the heat.

After it's cooled a bit, strain the mixture into a normal glass bowl. After the mixture has completely cooled, add the honey and continue to stir. Pour the syrup into a clean, sealable jar.

Take ½ tsp. to 1 tsp. a day for a child and 1 tbsp. a day for adults to ward off diseases; in the event of a cold or flu, take the dose every three hours.

ECHINACEA

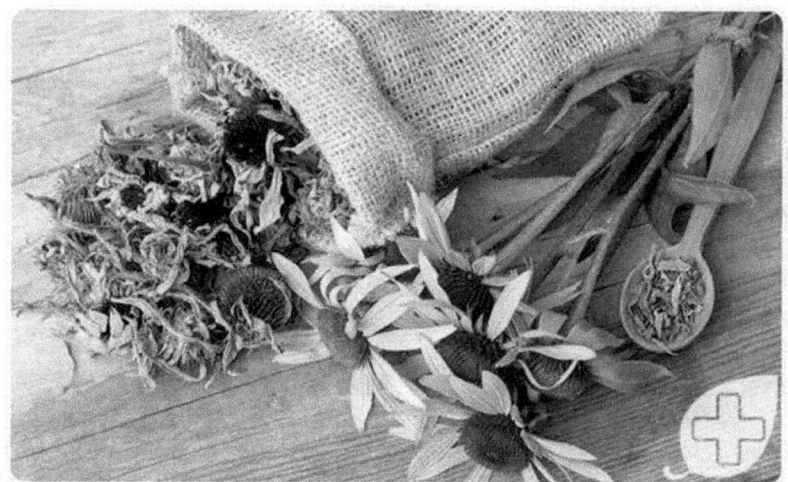

Immune system-boosting, beautiful purple-flower Echinacea has been shown to have essential antiviral abilities. The roots and the flowers of the Echinacea reduce the length and pain of the typical upper respiratory tract infection and the common cold. One must begin the Echinacea intake early so as to eliminate drastic symptoms.

Echinacea Root Tincture

Note: Echinacea tincture is perfect to eliminate early cold and flu symptoms. It doesn't taste great. Most people drip tiny amounts of the liquid into cups of water and take it that way. Regardless, Echinacea tincture is a vital herbal medicine.

Ingredients:
1 clean jar
40 proof vodka
Dried Echinacea root ***Directions:***
Begin by filling the jar you've chosen about ¾ full with the dried Echinacea root. Next, pour the vodka into the jar until the root is covered by approximately two inches. Place the lid on the jar and label the jar. Allow the jar to rest, sealed, in a dark cupboard for six weeks. About once a week, if you remember, shake the jar.

After six weeks, strain the herbs and keep the alcohol liquid. Pour this liquid into a small, sterile bottle. Dropper bottles work the best. Drop the tincture on the tongue in order to feel the tingling sensation of the Echinacea. The mixture should last two years.

Echinacea Antiviral Tea

Ingredients:
1 tbsp. lemon grass 1 tbsp. spearmint leaves 4 tbsp. Echinacea grounds (of roots, flowers, and leaves) 3 cups water

Directions:
Bring the three cups of water to boil over the stovetop. After it begins to boil, pour in the lemon grass, spearmint leaves, and the Echinacea grounds. Turn down the heat to low and allow the tea to simmer for thirty minutes. Afterwards, strain the tea and drink warm. The tea can keep in the refrigerator for three days.

GARLIC

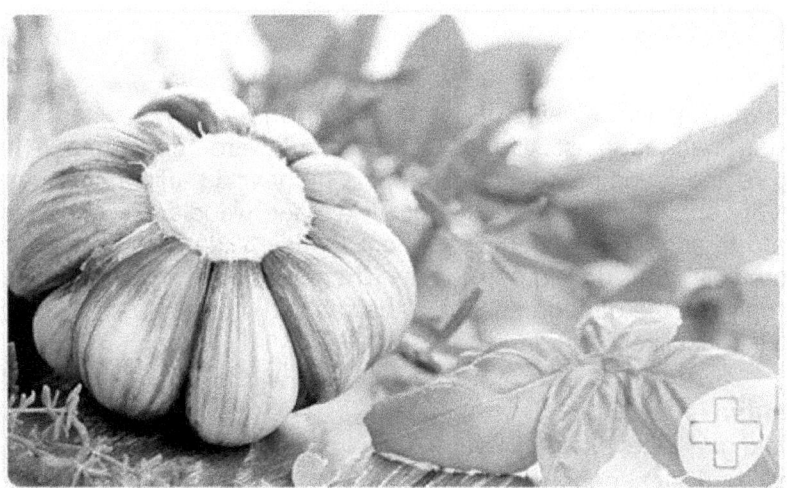

Garlic, that tasty herb, finds its home in spaghetti sauces and, yes, the medicine cabinet. It boosts the immune system and works to inhibit the reproductive rate of the viruses pulsing in the body. This is because garlic contains allicilin, a complex compound that can kill and inhibit the viruses.

Wild Garlic Pesto

The purported health benefits of garlic for both the immune system and for fighting back against viruses and bacteria are staggering. The following recipe recommends foraging for a bit of wild garlic that usually grows every spring at the very exterior of average woodlands. The plant is not hard to spot. The white flowers host a garlic scent; the plants also have incredibly long, dark green leaves. If suspicious about a particular plant, simply rub the dark green leaf. If the rubbing emits the garlic scent, the plant is most likely wild garlic.

Ingredients:
2 cups wild garlic leaves and flowers 200 ml olive oil
40 grams sunflower seeds ½ cup parsley
Salt and pepper to taste *Directions:*
Begin by boiling a cup of water. Blanch the garlic leaves in the boiling water for a full fifteen seconds. Immediately afterwards, rinse the leaves in cold water. Pat the leaves dry carefully. Place the leaves in a blender or a food processor along with the oil and the shelled sunflower seeds. Enjoy the wild garlic pesto.

Garlic Skin Treatment

Note: This ointment brings the viral and bacterial-fighting powers to the exterior body. It's perfect for rashes and cuts.

Ingredients:
3 tbsp. olive oil
3 tbsp. coconut oil (unrefined)
1 tbsp. crushed garlic

Directions:
Begin by placing the unrefined coconut oil in a small saucepan. Allow it to melt on low. Afterwards, pour in the three tablespoons of olive oil. Stir while they assimilate together. Remove the saucepan from the heat and add in the tablespoon of garlic. Pour the mixture into a food processor or blender, and blend the mixture together for two minutes.

Strain the liquid and place it in a sealable jar. Keep the jar in the refrigerator. The mixture will turn to a creamy ointment-like mixture in just one hour.

Rub the mixture on the skin for rashes, to fight candida, or to fight infection.

Rub the mixture on the chest for pneumonia and chest colds; rub it on the throat for colds and sore throats. Utilize it to cleanse one's self and eliminate bacteria and viruses anywhere on the body.

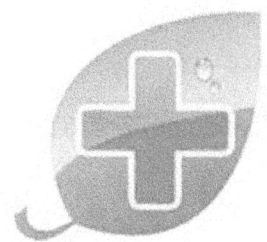

Chapter 5
ANTIBACTERIAL HERBS

CRANBERRY

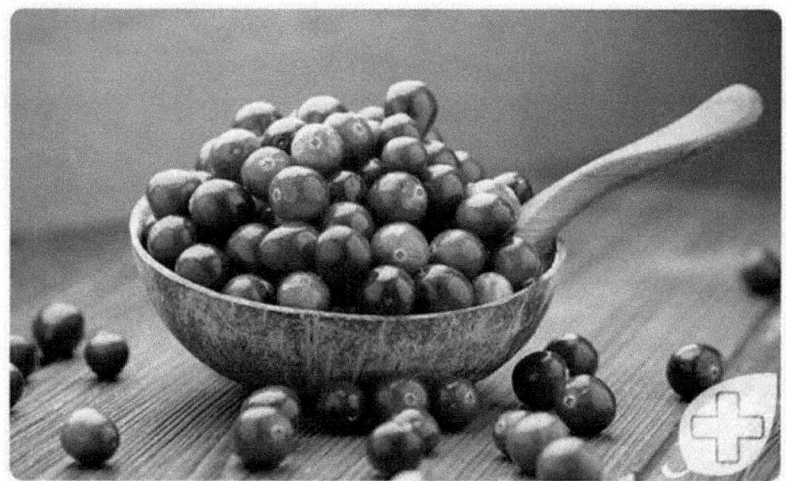

Cranberries have been shown to interfere with the bacteria in the lining of the bladder in women prone to bladder infections: sexually active women, pregnant women, and mature women. The bladder infection is caused after the bacteria have attached to the lining of the bladder. However, with the utilization of the cranberries, the bacteria can clear quickly and find no access to the kidneys.

Homemade Cranberry Juice

Ingredients:
8 cups water
½ cup agave nectar ½ cup fresh lemon juice ½ cup fresh orange juice 8 cups fresh cranberries ***Directions:***
Begin by bringing together the cranberries and the water in a large pot. Bring the cranberries to a boil and then turn the heat to low. Place a cover on the pot and allow it to simmer for a full thirty minutes.

Afterwards, bring the mixture into a food processor or blender. The mixture might have to be done bits at a time. Afterwards, add the agave nectar to the mixture along with the two fresh juices.

Place a sieve over a bowl and pour the juice overtop the sieve, make sure to collect.

Not-Just-Thanksgiving Cranberry Sauce

Ingredients:

12 ounces fresh or frozen cranberries

¾ cup sugar

1 cup water

Directions:

Bring together the water and the sugar in a medium-sized saucepan. Bring the water to a boil and pour in the cranberries. Allow the water to boost back to a boil. When this occurs, reduce the heat and allow the mixture to simmer for ten minutes. Continue to stir. Afterwards, cover the mixture and cool it outside of the refrigerator.

TEA TREE

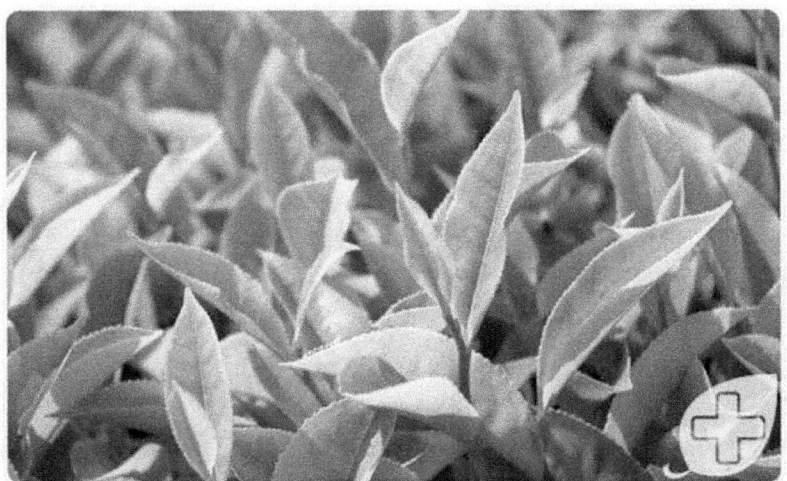

This Australian tree holds essential oil that works as an incredible antimicrobial agent when applied topically. It refutes the yeast called Candida albicans and the bacteria that causes the staph infection. Furthermore, people often utilize tea tree oil to treat fungal nail infections. Once tea tree oil is applied topically, the infection has been shown to improve dramatically.

Tea Tree Oil Ointment

Note: Utilize the following ointment topically in order to refute topical infection.

Ingredients:
4 ounces olive oil
2 ounces beeswax
40 drops lavender oil
20 drops tea tree oil

Directions:
Begin by melting the beeswax in a double boiler. Allow the wax to melt slowly. Afterwards, remove the beeswax from the double boiler and stir well. As the beeswax begins to cool, add the olive oil, the lavender oil, and the tea tree oil.

Store the ointment in a clean, sealable jar and apply topically in order to heal cuts and reduce infection.

Lice Reduction

When looking to eliminate head lice, drip a few drops of tea tree oil into shampoo and scrub the head with it. This should eliminate and prevent future lice attacks.

Natural Tea Tree Toothpaste

Ingredients:
1 tsp. sage
5 drops tea tree oil
4 tbsp. baking soda
3 tbsp. coconut oil

Directions:
Bring all the ingredients together in a small bowl and stir well. Place the mixture on a toothbrush and brush the teeth for approximately two minutes. Rinse the mouth with clean water.

ARTEMISIA

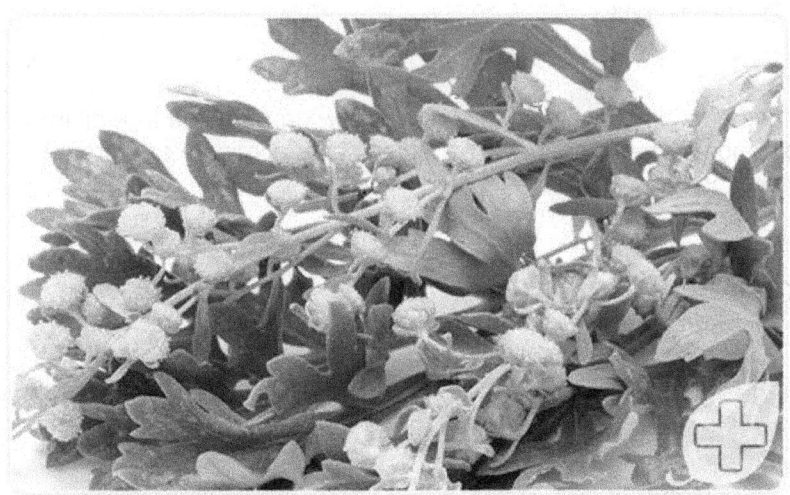

Asian-oriented Artemisia is a systemic herbal medicine. This means that it works through the bloodstream to administer health and strength to the bodily cells. Its active ingredient, artemisinin, works against strains of staphylococcus aureus, malaria, liver disease, cancer, MRSA, and epilepsy. There are several different Artemisia family members including sagebrush, mugwort, Tarragon, wormwood, and sagewort.

Tarragon Garlic Chicken

Ingredients:
½ tsp. dried tarragon
2 tsp. fresh tarragon
2 tsp. garlic oil
2 scallions
2 chicken breasts
½ tsp. salt
½ cup cream
1/3 cup white wine

Directions:
Place the garlic oil in a skillet and heat the oil on a medium-high setting. To the side, slice and dice the fresh tarragon and the scallions. Place the scallions and the dried tarragon in the garlic oil and stir for one minute.

Afterwards, place the chicken breasts in the skillet as well. Cook for five minutes. Be careful not to allow the scallions to burn on the bottom of the pan.

Next, flip the chicken breasts and pour in the white wine. Toss in the salt and place the lid overtop the skillet. Lower the heat to a low setting and allow it to simmer for ten minutes.

Remove the chicken from the skillet. Bring the leftover skillet mixture to a boil and pour in the cream. Continue to stir. Add the fresh tarragon pieces and stir. Salt and pepper overtop, as well.

Pour this tarragon-rich sauce over the chicken breasts. Add a bit more tarragon for extra health benefits, if desired.

Drink Absinthe

Absinthe is actually created with Artemisia absinthium, which is the technical term for wormwood. Drink absinthe for desired Artemisia properties.

USNEA

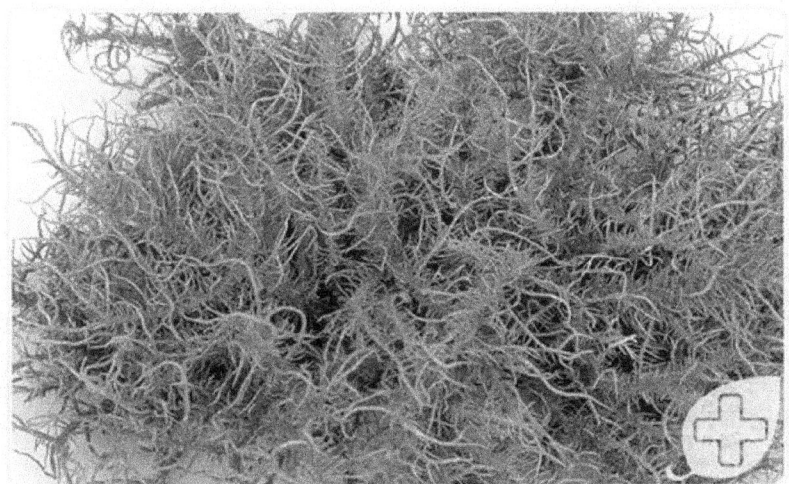

Natural formations of usnea can be found hanging from tree branches. This lichen's main ingredient is usnic acid, which targets gram-positive bacterium. Therefore, it leaves all good bacteria in the gut, thus allowing the immune system to strengthen rather than fail with the occurrence of a shortage of good flora. This usnic acid works to disrupt the bacteria's metabolic functions, thus forcing them to die.

Usnea Tincture

Ingredients:
Usnea herbs
Everclear
Water

Directions:
Begin by taking a glass mason jar and filling it three quarters of the way full with Usnea herbs. Afterwards, pour the Everclear overtop the herbs until you've topped it over two inches higher than the herbs. Pour a bit of water to fill the jar completely, and top the jar. Place the jar in a cool, dark location for six weeks.

Afterwards, strain the liquid and place the tincture in a small dropper. One can utilize the tincture by dripping it into cups of water or simply dropping a morsel on the tongue.

OREGANO

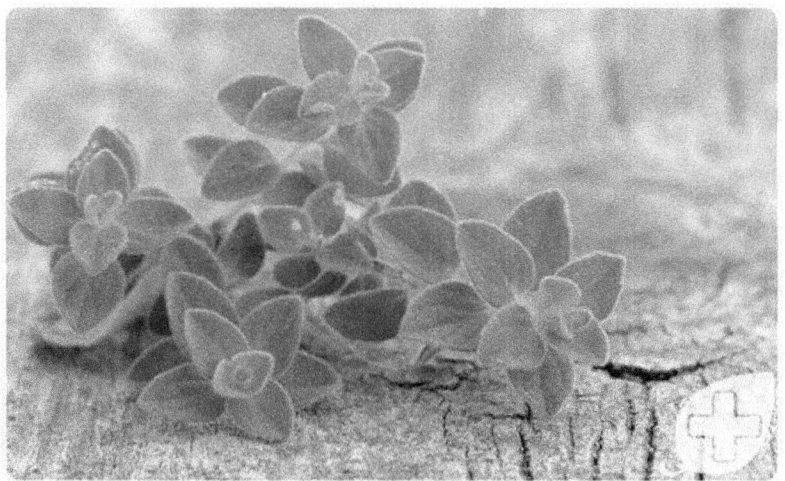

Mediterranean-native oregano is a world-renowned antibacterial herb. Its most active ingredient, carvacol, has been shown to be stronger than Streptomycin, penicillin, and one of the most powerful synthetic antibiotics, vancomycin. Oregano is a broad-usage antibiotic; it will therefore eliminate any sort of bacteria it approaches.

Oregano Tea

Drinking oregano tea offers wonderful assistance for those suffering from bacterial infections. Remember that oregano tea can have a bitter taste to it, one that can be rectified with a bit of honey.

Ingredients:
8 ounces water
1 ½ tsp. oregano leaves 1 tsp. honey

Directions:
Begin by bringing all eight ounces of water to boil in a small saucepan. After the water begins to boil, add the oregano immediately to the water and remove the water from the heat. Allow the oregano to steep in the water for a full five minutes. Afterwards, strain the tea and add honey, if desired. Enjoy.

Oregano Oil

Oregano oil works to alleviate pain, even when applied topically. Furthermore, breathing in the scent of the oil works to reduce nose and throat constriction and congestion. It further kills exterior bacteria and fungi.

Ingredients:
½ cup olive oil
½ cup oregano leaves

Directions:
Begin by preparing the oregano leaves. They should be fresh, rinsed and completely chopped.

Pour the olive oil into a clean glass jar along with the oregano leaves. To the side, bring a pot of water to a boil and place the clean glass jar in the boiling water. Allow the jar to rest in the hot water for ten minutes. Afterwards, remove the jar from the water and seal it. Place the jar on a window that receives a lot of sunlight. Allow it to sit for two weeks, shaking it every few days.

After the two weeks have passed, strain the oil and toss the leaves. Place the prepared oregano oil in a cleansed jar, and store the jar somewhere dark and cool.

MINT

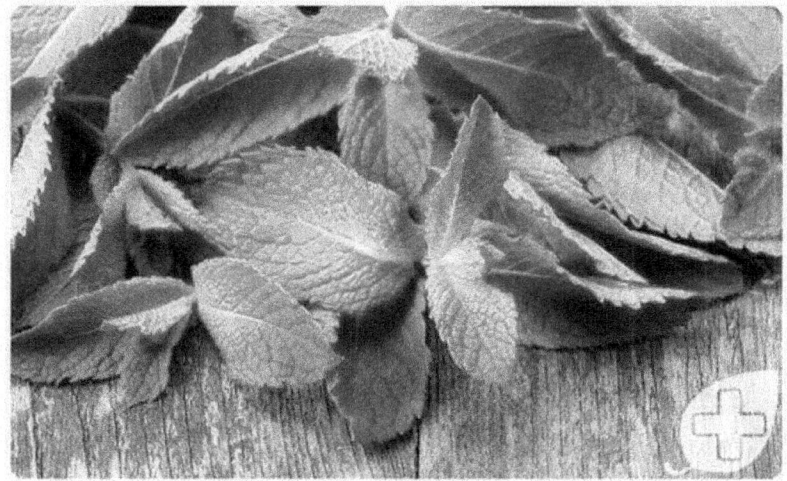

The mint family offers up a medical counter, as well, with a host of antibacterial effects. Look to thyme, sage, rosemary, lavender, basil, peppermint, and spearmint. Create a tea with any of the herbs: especially peppermint, spearmint, and sage.

CULINARY SPICES

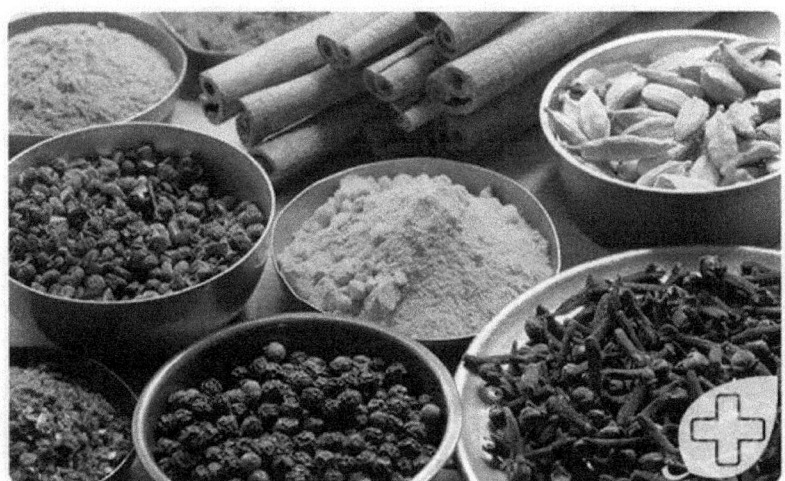

Further spices work to enhance the antimicrobial properties of foods, boosting the immune system and working against the harmful bacteria in the body. Look to cinnamon, clove, chilli peppers, nutmeg, horseradish, tamarind, and cumin.

Garlic and Cumin Hummus

Ingredients:
4 garlic cloves
1/3 cup olive oil
2 tsp. cumin
3 tbsp. tahini
2 cans chickpeas
1 tbsp. soy sauce
3 tbsp. lemon juice
½ tsp. salt

Directions:
Begin by slicing up the garlic cloves. Next, bring the olive oil and the sliced garlic together in a saucepan. Allow them to cook together for three minutes on medium. After three minutes, remove the pan from the heat and allow the pan to cool.

Next, place tahini, chickpeas, soy sauce, lemon juice, and salt in the food processor. Fish out the pieces of garlic from the saucepan and add them to the processor, as well. Keep the oil in the saucepan. Run the processor for twenty seconds. Afterwards, start to slowly pour in the cumin. After adding the cumin, slowly add the oil, as well. Continue to process until you've reached desired consistency. Enjoy.

Preparation of Herbs

The above herbs were linked with very specific recipes for utilization, for digesting and for strengthening the immune system. However, the preparation of herbs can be very general and is outlined below.

1. Dry the Herbs
When drying the herbs, harvest the herbs in the late summer. Cut the branches after exterior dew has evaporated. Do not gather any diseased, yellow branches. Hang these herbs upside down in a warm room and check on them once or twice a week until they've completely dried.

2. Store Dried Herbs
Always store the dried herbs in sealable, air-tight containers. Date the containers, and place them in a dry place.

3. Make a Tea or Infusion
Use boiled water and steep the herbs in the boiling water. Allow the herbs to steep for a full five minutes prior to straining the tea and drinking.

4. Make a Poultice
A poultice is a hot, wet mixture that is applied topically. Take the dried herbs and mix them with water until it creates a paste. Spread this paste on the skin and place a piece of gauze overtop the poultice and hold it in place.

5. Cook, Make an Essential Oil, and Include Many Herbs in Everyday Life
The herbs listed above can be included in everyday recipes, in everyday topical creams. Enjoy the benefits of the natural world and the wonderful flavours the herbs bring to each recipe.

Conclusion

The medical world of constant synthetic drugs is coming to a nasty halt. Instead of allowing greater and greater bacteria to evolve via the utilization of synthetic drugs, look to the earth, to the natural, herbal antibiotics. Each herb outlined in this book holds unique properties to boost the immune system, to refute viruses, and to beat back against bacteria. Rejuvenate the body and feel at one with the earth. Make confident, precise decisions about the unique, evolved plants that enter the body as antibiotics in tincture, tea, or food formation. Enjoy the wonderful flavors that build greater interior bodily strength. Hold antibiotics to a higher standard and understand the history of feeling well.

www.ingramcontent.com/pod-product-compliance
Lightning Source LLC
Chambersburg PA
CBHW071123030426
42336CB00013BA/2181